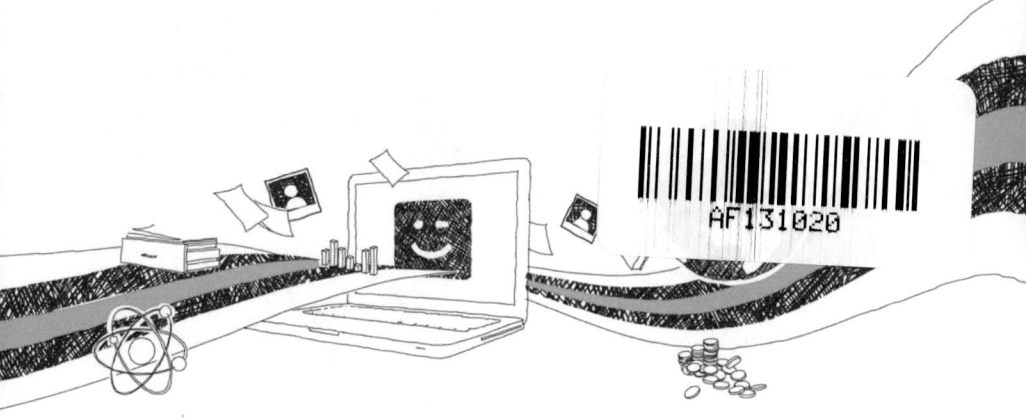
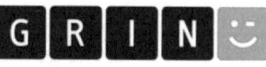

Bibliographic information published by the German National Library:

The German National Library lists this publication in the National Bibliography; detailed bibliographic data are available on the Internet at http://dnb.dnb.de .

Imprint:

Copyright © 2018 GRIN Verlag
Print and binding: Books on Demand GmbH, Norderstedt Germany
ISBN: 9783668626881

This book at GRIN:

https://www.grin.com/document/388313

Patrick Kimuyu

The Molecular Basis of Apoptosis

GRIN Verlag

GRIN - Your knowledge has value

Since its foundation in 1998, GRIN has specialized in publishing academic texts by students, college teachers and other academics as e-book and printed book. The website www.grin.com is an ideal platform for presenting term papers, final papers, scientific essays, dissertations and specialist books.

Visit us on the internet:

http://www.grin.com/

http://www.facebook.com/grincom

http://www.twitter.com/grin_com

The Molecular Basis of Apoptosis

Name: Patrick Kimuyu

Abstract

Apoptosis refers to a programmed cell death; a biological process in which the body of an organism destroys its cells for different reasons. In reality, apoptosis and necrosis involve different mechanisms, and this implies they are different. In addition, the changes that occur in the process of cell death are differing in terms of morphology and chemical composition.

Evidence indicates that there are various factors that make cells commit suicide. In most cases, cells commit suicide due to imbalances between positive and negative signals that determine cell survival. Cells can consider committing suicide upon the recipient of negative signals.

This research will provide a comprehensive overview of apoptosis. It will discuss mechanisms of apoptosis and the factors involved in the process. It will also explain the association between apoptosis.

Introduction

Apoptosis refers to a biological process in which the body of an organism destroys its cells for different reasons. Elmore (2007) defines apoptosis as a process that "occurs normally during development and aging and as a homeostatic mechanism to maintain cell populations in tissues" (p. 496). On the other hand, apoptosis occurs in other biological processes such as immune reactions and disease responses. As such, it plays a pivotal role in the body's defense mechanism. In reality, apoptosis is usually triggered by an array of stimuli and conditions including pathological and physiological factors. However, it is worth noting that, these stimuli may not necessarily cause death to all cells that receive the same stimulus owing to other biological signals that inhibit apoptosis in some cells while exposing others to programmed cell suicide. Stimuli that trigger apoptosis are diverse, and their mechanisms of cell death are different too. For instance, some stimuli can trigger cell death by apoptosis, whereas others trigger cell death by necrosis. These are distinct cell death processes, even though apoptosis is mostly confused with necrosis. Elmore (2007) states "It is the type of stimuli that determine if cells die by apoptosis or necrosis; a variety of injurious stimuli such as heat, radiation, hypoxia and cytotoxic anticancer drugs can induce apoptosis, but these same stimuli can result in necrosis at higher doses" (p. 497). Ordinarily, stimuli that cause DNA damage in cells trigger the process of apoptosis in which the cells are programmed to die through a cascade of cell death pathways. This process is referred to as 'programmed cell death' because it is an energy-dependent and coordinated process that involves "a complex cascade of events that link the initiating stimuli to the final demise of the cell" (Elmore, 2007 p.497). Therefore, this research paper will provide an overview on the process of apoptosis.

Distinguishing Apoptosis from Necrosis

Apoptosis is believed to be an alternative to necrosis; an energy-dependent mode of cell death involving a toxic process to degrade cells. However, it is worth noting that, apoptosis and necrosis involve different mechanisms, and this implies they are different. In addition, the changes that occur in the process of cell death are differing in terms of morphology and chemical composition.

From a distinctive approach, necrosis can be defined as cell death by injury in which cells experience mechanical damage or they are exposed to toxic chemicals leading to DNA damage. In necrosis, cell death exhibits a characteristic array of changes. For instance, the injured cells or organelles such as the mitochondria swell. This swelling is caused by the disruption of water and ions passage across the cell membrane. As a result, cytoplasmic cell contents leak out from the cell leading to a characteristic inflammation of the tissues surrounding the injury. In contrast, cell death by suicide (apoptosis) exhibits diverse changes in which cells are induced to undergo suicide. The processes involved in apoptosis are orderly in which the cell shrinks to initiate apoptotic cascades until the cell exposes the 'eat me' signal on the cell membrane to facilitate binding with phagocytes (Edmonds, 2010). In turn, phagocytes are induced to produce anti-inflammatory agents such as TGF-β and IL-10; thus inflammation does not occur in apoptosis.

Despite the morphological and mechanism differences exhibited by apoptosis and necrosis, there is a significant overlap between these processes. It is evident that apoptosis and necrosis "represent morphologic expressions of a shared biochemical network described as the "apoptosis-necrosis continuum" (Zeiss, 2003 p. 493).

Factors Leading to Cell Suicide

Evidence indicates that there are various factors that make cells commit suicide. In most cases, cells commit suicide due to imbalances between positive and negative signals that determine cell survival. Ordinarily, positive signals control the biological processes of the cells, whereas negative signals impair cellular activity. Therefore, a transient balance between these signals is necessary for cell survival or death. In most cases, cells commit suicide when positive signals are withdrawn implying that some processes that sustain survival are interrupted; thus, the cell cannot continue with its biological processes. As a result, the cell decides to commit suicide. Some of the most significant positive signals are growth factors for neurons and Interleukin-2 (IL-2). IL-2 signal plays a pivotal role in the mitosis of lymphocytes; thus, its withdrawal disrupts cell functioning.

On the other hand, cells can consider committing suicide upon the recipient of negative signals. In most cases, negative signals are generated when the synthesis of functional proteins is impaired leading to the production of defective proteins that lack the tertiary structure. In addition, negative signals are generated when oxidants accumulate within the cell leading to DNA damage. As a result, cell death activators including lymphotoxin, *Fas* ligand (*FasL*) and Tumor necrosis factor-alpha (TNF-α) initiate the apoptosis program (Elmore, 2007). Some of the agents that can lead to the generation of negative signals are X-rays, ultraviolet light and chemotherapeutic drugs.

Mechanisms of Apoptosis

Mechanisms of apoptosis are known to be highly sophisticated and complex owing to the series of molecular events that are energy-dependent. To date, there are three principal pathways through which apoptosis occur in the cells. These pathways are defined depending on the sources of the signals involved in triggering programmed cell suicide. These pathways are extrinsic (also known as death receptor pathway), intrinsic (mitochondrial) pathway and the Perforin/granzyme Pathway that involves the apoptosis-inducing factor (AIF). Despite the distinctive nature of these pathways, primary regarding the sources of their signals, these pathways converge at the final process that is defined as the terminal (execution) pathway through which cells are cellular contents are degraded. However, it is worth noting that, both extrinsic and intrinsic pathways are linked in some ways. Elmore reports "there is now evidence that the two pathways are linked and that molecules in one pathway can influence the other" (p. 514).

Extrinsic Pathway

Extrinsic signaling pathway is usually triggered by external signals, and it involves changes on the integral membrane proteins on the cells' plasma membrane. As such, extrinsic pathway can be described as receptor-mediated pathway because it involves cytotoxic T cells. Some of the main receptors involved in the extrinsic pathway are TNF and *Fas* receptors, and their binding forms a complementary death activator that transmits signals to the cell cytoplasm (Elmore, 2007). These signals send to the cytoplasm by the death activator leads to the activation of caspase 8. In turn, caspase 8 initiates molecular events involved in caspase activation leading to the engulfing of the cell by macrophages through phagocytosis. Ordinarily, cytotoxic T cells bind to their targets and expose *Fas*L on the cell surface. The intensity of *Fas*L produced on the cell surface depends on the intensity of the stimuli. Thereafter, *Fas* receptors bind with *Fas*L,

6

and this initiates cell death by apoptosis. However, it is worth noting that, the binding of *Fas* receptor and *Fas*L destines the cell for the execution pathway.

Intrinsic Pathway

Intrinsic pathway is controlled by internal signals from the mitochondria. As such, it is a non-receptor mediated pathway. Evidence indicates that, intracellular signals act as negative or positive signals that initiate mitochondria-related events. Cells exhibit death suppression programs that ensure cell survival, and these programs involve the production of cytokines, hormones and growth factors. Therefore, intrinsic pathway involves negative signals leading to the loss of apoptotic suppression and withdrawal of the main factors involved in the suppression of death programs.

The mechanism of the intrinsic pathway begins with the migration of *Bax* protein to the mitochondrial surface where it binds with Bcl-2; the protein that inhibits apoptosis, and causes the leakage of *cytochrome c*. *Cytochrome c* binds to the Apoptotic protease activating factor-1 (Apaf-1) and form apoptosome complexes. These complexes activate caspase 9 that releases proteases to cleave cellular proteins.

Perforin/Granzyme Pathway

This pathway involves CD8+ cells that destroy antigen-bearing cells by apoptosis. Evidence shows that, perforin/granzyme pathway is a variant pathway for Type IV hypersensitivity in which cells T-cell mediated toxicity occur. Ordinarily, *Fas*L/*Fas*R proteins interact to cause CTL-induced apoptosis (Brunner et al., 2003). In this pathway, Apoptosis-inducing factor is released from the inter-membrane space of the mitochondria, and it migrates to the nucleus where it binds with DNA to trigger cell death by apoptosis. This pathway uses a different mechanism from the other two pathways to initiate apoptosis by using neurons, rather than caspases.

Execution Pathway

Execution pathway completes the process of apoptosis in which active caspases lead to the activation of cytoplasmic endonucleases and proteases. Endonucleases degrade nuclear materials, whereas cytoplasmic proteases degrade the cytoskeletal and nuclear proteins. In this pathway, caspases (Caspase-3, caspase-6 and caspase-7) acts as executor caspases in which various cellular components are cleaved leading to biochemical and morphological changes observed in apoptotic cells (Elmore, 2007). This pathway is followed by the uptake of the cells by phagocytes, and this is believed to be the final process of apoptosis.

Reasons for Programmed Cell Death

From a biological perspective, apoptosis occurs for two main reasons. The first one is controlling developmental processes in the body of an organism. This is referred to as physiologic apoptosis. Secondly, apoptosis occurs to destroy cells that compromise the integrity of an organism. This form of programmed cell death occurs in what is referred to as pathologic apoptosis because; it responds to pathogens that cause harm to the organism.

Physiologic Apoptosis

In physiologic apoptosis, cell death occurs to regulate the population of various cells by demonstrating a complementary opposite role to that of mitosis and cell proliferation. This is the reason physiologic apoptosis is considered as important as the mitosis process in various developmental processes. Elmore states "Apoptosis is critically important during various developmental processes; as examples, both the nervous system and the immune system arise through overproduction of cells" (p. 510). He adds "apoptosis is central to remodeling in the adult, such as the follicular atresia of the post ovulatory follicle and post-weaning mammary gland involution, to name a couple of examples' (p. 510).

Concisely, apoptosis plays significant roles in the development of various organisms. For instance, the process of metamorphosis in both insects and tadpoles occur through apoptosis. In insects, the development from the pupal stage to an adult stage involves apoptosis in which some cells die through apoptosis to generate nutrients required for the development of some structures of the adult insect. On the other hand, tadpoles undergo metamorphosis to the adult stage through apoptosis in which the tail is reabsorbed as the tadpole advances into the adult stage (Renehan et al 1537). This is why adult frogs do not have tails, and yet their precursors posses tails.

Another developmental process in which apoptosis plays significant roles is during embryonic development of organisms. For instance, the formation of fingers and toes in the fetuses of animals including humans involves the removal of cells between the digits by apoptosis. Ordinarily, the formation of the limbs results into webbed palms or feet, after which cells between the fingers or toes die off by apoptosis.

Moreover, the formation of synapses between neurons in the nervous system requires apoptosis. In this process, surplus cells that are adjacent to the synapses cleft are removed to create synaptic junctions between neurons through which neurotransmitters are conveyed during impulse transmission.

Pathologic Apoptosis

Pathologic apoptosis occurs to regulate cell death in some diseases such as cancer, AIDS, autoimmune lymphoproliferative syndrome, ischemia and amyotrophic lateral sclerosis. However, it is worth noting that, the extent of apoptosis depends on the condition present in which some conditions trigger extensive apoptosis, whereas others are associated with insignificant apoptosis. For instance, neurodegenerative diseases, ischemia-associated injury and autoimmune diseases exhibit excessive apoptosis.

There are various situations through which pathologic apoptosis occur. The first example of pathologic apoptosis is associated with viral infection in which cytotoxic T lymphocytes are activated to initiate extrinsic pathway for apoptosis. By carrying out apoptosis of virus-infected cells, the body gets rid of the viruses; thus, preventing their pathogenicity which is manifested as a disease condition. On the other hand, apoptosis occurs in cell-mediated immune responses in which effector cells are removed from the body before they attack body constituents. Ordinarily, cell-mediated immune responses play pivotal roles in preventing the destruction of 'self' proteins, this is why autoimmune diseases such as rheumatoid arthritis (RA) and systemic lupus erythematosus (SLE) occur, owing to defects in the cellular proteins, primary those involved in the apoptosis machinery.

On the other hand, pathologic apoptosis occurs on cells with DNA damage. In most cases, DNA damage leads to gene mutations that disrupt embryonic development of organisms. This leads to birth defects in offsprings or the development of cancerous cells, especially in adult organisms. In such circumstances, the cells produce *p53* protein that induces apoptosis. This implies that, mutations in *p53* gene lead to devastating consequences including the development of cancer (Gu et al., 2001).

Apoptosis and Cancer

Apoptosis is related to some cancers that are caused by viruses such as the Human Papilloma Virus (HPV) and Epstein-Barr virus (EBV). These viruses produce proteins such as E6 to inhibit *p53* that acts as the main apoptosis promoter gene. As such, these viruses transform

10

human cells and prevent apoptosis leading to the development of lymphomas. Burkitt lymphoma is an outstanding example of virus-caused lymphoma in which apoptosis is inhibited.

It is also believed that, EBV inhibits the activity of tumor suppressor genes of B-lymphocytes because it produces some proteins which possess anti-apoptotic properties. For instance, EBV-encoded RNAs and EBV nuclear antigen-1 (EBNA-1) inhibit apoptosis process in lymphoid tissues. On the other hand, BCL-2 protein in lymphocytes which act as anti-apoptotic agent during cell proliferation is inhibited by EBNA-3C AND EBNA-3A produced by Epstein-Barr virus leading to the transformation of normal lymphocytes into cancerous cells (Kanbar et al., 2014).

Moreover, *C-myc oncogene* activation in Burkitt lymphoma is believed to be caused by reciprocal gene translocations between chromosome 8 and 14. Chromosome 2 and 22 are also involved in these translocations which cause the activation of *C-myc oncogene*s. Research shows that, 80% of Burkitt lymphoma is caused by translocation t (8; 14) in which *C-myc oncogene* on chromosome 8 undergoes transposition on chromosome 14 resulting into the activation of *C-myc oncogene*, which is responsible for tumor proliferation in the lymphoid tissue. On the other hand, translocation *t (8; 2)* and *t (8; 22)* causes gene changes in chromosome 2, primarily on the kappa light chain of the immunoglobulin (Hudson, Link & Weinstein, 2007). Therefore, gene changes in immunoglobulin chains lead to the activation of *C-myc oncogene*s involved in the transformation of normal lymphocytes into tumor cells. Activation of *C-myc oncogene*s leads to the overproduction of C-myc proteins, which influence the expression of *p53* gene and DAP-kinase. These two products are involved in cell apoptosis in which they slow down the process of cell division. C-myc proteins are also believed to act as transcription factors during the cell cycle, including differentiation, growth, adhesion and apoptosis. Research indicates that, C-myc

11

gene overexpression leads to the induction of *TRAP1*, *cyclin D2* and *HLA-DRB1* genes while PDGFR-alpha production is repressed leading to the formation of lymphomas (Kanbar et al., 2014).

Inhibition of Apoptosis

Inhibition of apoptosis does not occur in pathologic apoptosis only, but also some biological processes in various sites of the body. For instance, antigens in the so-called 'immunologically privileged sites' such as the testes and the anterior chamber of the eye exhibit molecular events that inhibit apoptosis. The mechanism of preventing apoptosis in these sites is controlled by the expression of high levels of *Fas*L throughout the cell cycle. As a result, antigen-reactive T cells such as cytotoxic cells that express *Fas* are destroyed in these sites. In other words, these sites exhibit anti-apoptotic characteristics, and this implies that graft rejection in organ transplants can be prevented by the use of high levels of *Fas*L.

Conclusion

In a brief conclusion, apoptosis can be described as a biological process through which cells are destroyed in the body using its own mechanisms. It is referred to as programmed cell death because it involves an array of molecular events that are coordinated orderly. It differs from necrosis by cell morphology and biochemical properties. For instance, in apoptosis, inflammation does not occur, whereas this phenomenon is witnessed in necrosis.

Apoptosis is triggered by various stimuli including DNA damage by oxidants such as therapeutic drugs, X-rays and ultraviolet light. Evidence shows that, DNA damage causes the release of various chemicals and agents that serve as signals for cell death. In most cases, negative signals cause the disruption of protein synthesis processes leading to the activation of caspases by death activators.

In theory, external signals trigger extrinsic apoptosis in which cytotoxic T cells induce cell death cascades. On the other hand, internal signals trigger intrinsic apoptosis and this process is controlled by the mitochondria. These processes cause apoptosis for two main reasons; regulation of cell populations and the removal of pathogen-infected cells.

References

Brunner, T. et al. (2003). *Fas* (CD95/Apo-1) Ligand Regulation in T cell Homeostasis, Cell-mediated Cytotoxicity and Immune Pathology. *Semin Immunol.* 15:167–76.

Edmonds, M. (2010). *What is apoptosis?* Retrieved from http://science.howstuffworks.com/life/cellular-microscopic/apoptosis.htm

Elmore, S. (2007). Apoptosis: A Review of Programmed Cell Death. *Toxicol. Pathol.* 35(4): 495-516. Retrieved from http://www.ncbi.nlm.nih.gov/pmc/articles/PMC2117903/

Gu, J. et al. (2001). Mechanism of Functional Inactivation of a Li-Fraumeni Syndrome *P53* That has a Mutation Outside of the DNA-Binding Domain. *Cancer Res.*, 61:1741–6.

Hudson, M., Link, M. & Weinstein, H. (2007). *Pediatric Lymphomas.* New York, NY: Springer.

Kanbar, A. et al. (2014). *Burkitt Lymphoma and Burkitt-like Lymphoma.* Retrieved from http://emedicine.medscape.com/article/1447602-overview#showall

Renehan, G et al. (2001). What Is Apoptosis, and Why Is It Important? *BMJ.* 322:1536–8.

Zeiss, J. (2003). The Apoptosis-Necrosis Continuum: Insights from Genetically Altered Mice. *Vet Pathol.* 40:481–95.

YOUR KNOWLEDGE HAS VALUE

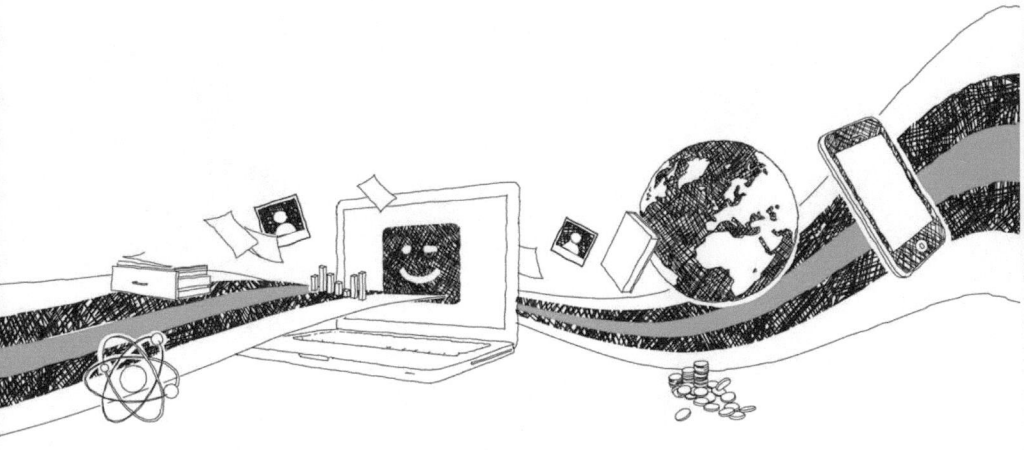

- We will publish your bachelor's and master's thesis, essays and papers

- Your own eBook and book - sold worldwide in all relevant shops

- Earn money with each sale

Upload your text at www.GRIN.com
and publish for free

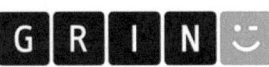